For my two beautiful girls...

let this be proof that anything is possible!

First published in 2019 through the
Independent Publishing Network (IPN)

ISBN 978-1-78972-727-2

No Dummy For Mummy

From Poppy Seed To Parrot

by Sally R. Wilkes

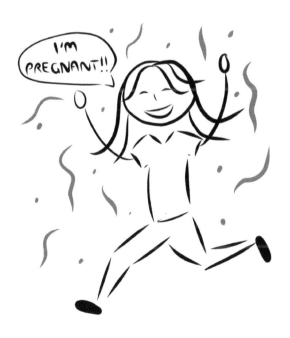

Introduction

I'm not entirely sure at what point I learnt to put on a front. Growing up in Yorkshire I would always hear phrases like "there's nowt that can't be solved with a cuppa" and "c'mon lass ya made a tougher stuff than that". So to be honest I don't ever remember truly opening up about how I felt. I've always been brilliant at spotting when friends and family are struggling but ask me how I'm doing..."I'm great, loving life, couldn't be better"...even if this is the polar opposite to how I'm feeling.

After the birth of my eldest daughter, I felt like I was drowning in emotions. I was overwhelmingly happy, proud and completely in love with her. But at the same time I was anxious, lonely and terrified that something horrible was going to happen. All these emotions were intensified by a prolonged sleep drought and I reached a point where I was struggling to hold up my iron wall. But I was too afraid to let it go and so, I battled on. So much so that many of my close friends and family reading this will probably be surprised to hear I was even struggling.

When my daughter was 10 weeks old, I picked up my phone and began to write things down in the notes section. I wrote little rhymes all about the good, the bad and the disgusting. To my surprise, I found that I actually had quite a talent. But not only that, I had found a way to release my emotions that didn't leave me feeling exposed. Three and a half years on I have learnt that I don't always have to be "strong". I look back at that time and want to shake myself for not just being more honest.

This book is a collection of rhymes written at my happiest and at my most vulnerable moments. It is in no way judgemental, simply an open and honest account of my parenting journey from pregnancy up until my eldest daughter turned two. If you're a parent reading this then I want you to know that you are not on your own. It's normal to find things difficult and there is no shame whatsoever in admitting that you are struggling!

Wish Upon A Wee

I'm watching the timer sat on the bathroom floor.

Trying not to get my hopes up as we've been here before.

Then with a sinking feeling, I pick up the stick.

Hang on a minute though. Is this a trick?

A very faint line has appeared on the display.

It's probably a fault. I'll just throw the test away.

But was it? Am I? What did that really mean?

I won't tell my husband, I don't want to make a scene.

That brand was quite a cheap one. Perhaps it's not the best.

I'll have to wait until the morning and buy another test.

So here I go again making a wish upon a wee.

But this time it says "PREGNANT" clear for all to see.

I fly down the stairs at cheetah lightning pace.

I find my hubby in the kitchen and wave it in his face.

"The test says that I'm pregnant" I start to jump and shout.

To which my hubby says "ha you will have to push it out!"

What a nice mature response! But I can not hide my grin.

I have a poppy seed inside me and adventures to begin!

I don't think I will ever forget the rollercoaster of emotions involved in trying for a baby. The journey starts with excitement, hope and a gazillion ideas in your head of what the future holds for you and your baby. For some fortunate people, this journey is a short one. For me, what followed was a transition to frustration, then worry and then to despair.

In comparison to many, our journey was a simple one. But I have never been the most patient person (cue laughter from my husband and my parents). Each month I would do a pregnancy test before I even knew whether my period was late. And each month the test was negative. I would cry then get annoyed at my husband because it hadn't "worked". Hardly the happy, loving picture I'd imagined when starting a family!

So when the test finally showed a very faint line, I was in disbelief. I was convinced it must be a faulty test so I didn't say anything to my husband. It was a Saturday morning so I made up some random reason why I needed to pop to the supermarket and went and bought two packs of early detection pregnancy kits. I went home and used them all in one go (which basically equates to pissing on £30 worth of cash, given how expensive those things are!)

Try Ginger

I'm definitely pregnant! My breakfast told me so.

Then my lunch and my dinner. There's nothing left to go!

"Try ginger" she says, "or a plain dry cracker."

If I didn't feel so crap, I'd probably just smack her.

I can't even keep an ice pop down. I just want to cry.

I think it's time to see the doctor to find out why.

"It's hyperemesis gravidarum. I'm prescribing you a pill."

But now I'm worried silly it will make the baby ill.

So I'll try to soldier on and ignore what he has said.

The baby comes first even though I feel half dead.

It took a while to see that I hadn't thought this through.

If I can't eat then the baby can't eat too.

But the tablets won't stay down so it's time for a jab.

"Remove your trousers please, it goes in your bum flab."

Oh my god that hurt but it's clearly done the trick.

For the first time I feel hungry instead of feeling sick!

At around six weeks pregnant, I began to feel rough...really rough. It started with a bit of nausea but rapidly spiralled out of control. Every morning I had a 30 to 40 minute commute to work and I had to take a plastic food container in the car with me, not to store my packed lunch, but to catch my partly digested breakfast mid drive. And it didn't stop with breakfast!

Two weeks later, I was walking in between sites at work and found myself bent over at the side of the road, unable to stop wretching and feeling like I was going to pass out. Not only did I feel horrific physically, I also felt like I was failing at being pregnant in some way. Writing this now, it seems like such a silly thing to feel. I called my husband who managed to get me straight in to see the doctor later that afternoon and he immediately diagnosed it as hyperemesis gravidarum.

We took photos of my bump every week throughout my pregnancy and from these it is clear to see that my stomach actually went in before it started expanding. And yet people were still quick to offer their "helpful" suggestions: "eat ginger biscuits or suck on a mint". IF ONLY!! I can honestly say that I have never known sickness like it!

A Fricking Melon

Before I fell pregnant, that was all I thought about.

But when I saw the plus sign...argh I'll have to push it out!

So as my belly grows, it's the birth that I now dwell on.

A raspberry I could cope with but it's now a fricking melon!

So we've signed up to some classes meant for parents-to-be.

And I'm so relieved to find that it isn't only me.

Six couples here in total all trying to figure out.

What birth and babies are really all about.

Our teacher is the best, she really can't do more.

She keeps us all smiling even talking blood and gore.

Our nerves are slowly easing and we all feel more prepared.

But best of all we know that our thoughts can now be shared.

I know that not everyone has positive things to say when it comes to antenatal classes. For me personally, had I not attended then I would have walked into parenthood in ignorant bliss and been in for the biggest shock of my life. I thought I was quite well informed when it came to birth and babies. I mean, I had watched endless episodes of One Born Every Minute so how could I not be!? Oh how wrong I was.

I knew nothing about the stages of labour or the choices available to me during labour. I knew nothing about how your milk comes in or that you bleed A LOT for quite some time after birth. And I knew nothing of how my mental health would be impacted. So the information provided during these classes was invaluable.

However, it was the group of mums I met through attending these classes that made the biggest difference for me. We were all going through the same things at the same time so could be there for each other in a way that no one else could be. The group has since disbanded but I will be forever grateful for the love and support I received from this group at such a life altering time. Our antenatal teacher was also brilliant and has continued to be a huge influence and support in my life. She is forever championing me and my work and I now consider her a very good friend.

The Birth Inquiry

Everybody pictures how they want their birth to be.

A simple, painless water birth was the birth I'd dreamt for me.

That didn't really go to plan, I was two weeks overdue.

And ready to do anything that I was told to do.

First they broke my waters, then they put me on a drip.

Then I nearly broke my husband's hand with my superhuman grip.

I couldn't hold a conversation, just the odd word said in slur.

To be honest, the rest of it is really quite a blur.

Our baby girl was born with some help along the way.

But all that really mattered was that we were both okay.

So when we felt ready, we began to share our news.

How much does she weigh? And what name did you choose?

Did you need pain relief? Gas and air or injection?

Did you push her out yourself or have a c-section?

Why's all that important? Giving birth is not a test!

To get that little baby out, you do whatever's best!

I'm not going to go into details but my birth was quite a traumatic experience. When our daughter finally arrived, I was so drugged up to the eyeballs that I don't really remember much of those first few hours with her. I finally came round and remember sitting up in my hospital bed on the ward holding this delicate, beautiful baby and my excitement began to build. We couldn't wait to share the news so we both decided on what we were going to say and sent out a message.

We soon started getting replies but what I hadn't prepared for was the number of people who came back asking whether I'd had a "natural" birth and whether I'd needed pain relief. I felt like I was being measured up against some sort of gold standard! Why does it matter what happened? And what's more, I was nowhere near ready to talk about the experience.

I'm all for being open when it comes to talking about birth as women need to have some idea of what is to come. But to those people who promote unrealistic expectations of birth...perhaps you should think carefully about the message you are sending to society. For the vast majority of women, birth is hard enough without being made to feel that you have failed at the end of it!

Just Milk Me

My baby girl is here, born just three days ago.

But it's not all smiles and roses, there's so much I didn't know.

First of all, I feel like I've been hit by a truck.

And these massive mama pads mean I'm waddling like a duck.

My bump once tight and firm is now a mass of jelly.

I'm sick of seeing the midwife, I just want to watch the telly.

My boobs are full to bursting, they're really hurting now.

I've pleaded with my husband to milk me like a cow.

Rewrite the truck...I was hit by a train!

Every time I feed my baby the contractions start again.

And oh my word the stitches, I've been really scared to poo.

So I've been eating figs and prunes like I'm the age of eighty-two.

But ask me if it's worth it, I'll say yes without a doubt.

This precious baby in my arms...she's what it's all about.

I don't think anyone or anything could have prepared me for post birth. I knew that I'd be tired, that was a given. And I didn't think for a minute that I would look as glamorous as the Duchess of Cambridge because I never do! But I had this extremely naive image of myself gliding out of hospital back in my normal clothes and heading home to resume daily life, but now with the added bonus of baby snuggles and pram walks. I know...what an idiot!

In actual fact, I left the hospital wearing men's pyjama bottoms and flip flops, shuffling across the car park with my legs as wide apart as they could go. I went home for all of three days before I was back in hospital with mastitis. I was fine one minute then crying the next for no apparent reason and I was going through more maternity pads than my baby was through nappies!

We went out for a short walk near our house and my husband marched ahead with the pram like the grand old Duke of flipping York whilst I trailed along behind with my boobs dragging me down and my arse in the air looking like some kind of elderly neanderthal. If you'd have painted this image and handed it to me pre birth, I would probably have told you to piss off!

Pop To The Shop

We've run out of milk and we need more bread.

It's okay, I'll just pop to the shop, I said.

I'll get our things together. It will only take a minute.

So I set up the pram and lay the baby in it.

She could do with a blanket. It's chilly out there.

And I need to pack the change bag with everything spare.

Wait a minute. Oh god, what's that smell!?

A quick change of her nappy and all is well.

Right, the pram needs a cover as it's started to rain.

Oh no she's crying, she's hungry again.

Another long feed then a quick wee for me.

I finally think we're ready, now where is my key!?

When you have a baby or a small child, there is no popping, nipping, dashing, or whizzing anywhere! Gone are the days of grabbing your keys and purse, and heading for the door. Try multiplying those two items by ten! Nappies, wipes, change mat, spare clothes, milk, snacks, toys, teethers, dummies...I've probably forgotten something even now!

If you ever want to get anywhere on time, you need to start planning your exit at least half an hour before you're due to leave. You first need to get a handle on the feed/poo cycle - if that is even possible! It is almost inevitable that the moment you lay them in their car seat or pushchair, you will be hit with a pungent smell! Either that or they will bring up their entire feed all down their clean clothes.

As a new mum, I found this whole process quite debilitating. It was like I'd completely lost my independence. I can completely understand how some parents lose their confidence and find themselves a prisoner in their own home. I was lucky enough to have a support network of other mums around me who would arrange meet ups at least twice a week during those early months which forced me to go out. Otherwise, it would have been so easy for me to retreat back into my house and never leave.

Just Ten Weeks

Just ten weeks since you came into my life.

You made me a mummy, no longer just a wife.

Ten tiny fingers, ten tiny toes.

Big brown eyes and a cute button nose.

A tiny baby held close to my chest.

Feeling overwhelmed and unbelievably blessed.

Just ten weeks to turn my world upside down.

It's mid afternoon and I'm still in my gown.

Covered in sick, wee and probably poo.

I haven't showered now for a day or two.

You're screaming, for what? I haven't a clue.

But it's okay, I'm your mummy, I love you.

Just ten weeks and you have everyone's attention.

Relatives, friends, even strangers have to mention.

Isn't she beautiful, oh look at her smile.

As they walk by your pram in the shopping aisle.

I try not to show but I'm incredibly smug.

You're all mine to keep, to kiss and to hug!

This is the rhyme that kick started this entire book. It had been a particularly bad night in terms of sleep. I can't remember why exactly as there have been many sleepless nights since then and they have all blurred into one! I was beyond exhausted and my husband had left early for work that morning so I'd been on my own for several hours with my daughter who just wouldn't stop screaming.

She didn't want feeding or winding, her nappy was dry, she didn't want putting down but she wouldn't settle in my arms either. Every parent has been there. It was getting close to lunchtime and I was still wearing my sick-stained dressing gown. Then all of a sudden, for no rhyme or reason (do you like what I've done there?), she stopped crying and fell asleep in my arms.

By this point I was ready to burst into tears. I readied myself to gently move her to the crib so that I could go and shower. But then I looked down at her peacefully sleeping in my arms and it all just washed away. The shower could wait. The housework could wait. There was no where else I needed to be. I sat there and enjoyed the cuddles and the quiet. Then I picked up my phone, opened the notes section and began to write.

Cough, Laugh, Leak

I have learnt so many things that I didn't know before.

One of these things is that I have a pelvic floor.

I'd never even heard this term at twenty-eight years old.

So I was a bit confused when pregnant to finally be told.

It's time to work on pelvic floors so sit down, let's begin.

Pretend you're desperate for a wee and you're trying to hold it in.

Now count to ten still holding, then slowly let it go.

Do this every single day, it will help with things below.

It's important that you carry on, even when you're baby-free.

Or you'll find that when you cough or laugh, you'll leak a little wee!

Yes it's true...I had no idea what a pelvic floor was, let alone that I had one myself! It's one of those things that no one had ever told me about and we certainly didn't learn about it at school. So when I fell pregnant and everyone started mentioning pelvic floors, I had absolutely no idea what they were talking about.

I think my midwife may have mentioned something in passing about pelvic floor exercises but she didn't go into detail and I didn't think to ask. So when I started attending pregnancy yoga classes and everyone was sitting there with a glazed look on their faces doing pelvic floor exercises, I wondered what the hell was going on. How do I exercise my pelvic floor when I don't even know how to find it!? Then one of the other women in the class came up with the most perfect analogy: imagine that you are sitting in a bathtub and an eel appears in the water. It swims towards you as though it's about to go inside you...what do you do? That's your pelvic floor!

There is a common misconception that only women who have a vaginal birth need to continue pelvic floor exercises once the baby is born. But regardless of whether you gave birth vaginally or through a c-section, you still had a melon sat on your bladder for several months. So if you don't fancy a leaky bladder then I'd really recommend keeping up with the exercises!

Losing The Plot

My husband thought me mad before, now I've "lost the plot".

I'm pulling faces in the mirror and dancing round the cot.

Saying mu mu mu mu mummy five hundred times a day.

She will NOT say daddy first, there's no way Jose!

A degree in mathematics yet I can't add two and two.

Shouting "it's okay I'm coming back" whilst sitting on the loo.

Making trump sounds with my mouth just walking down the street.

My boobs are out in public, there's no more being discreet.

There's a teabag in my sandwich...I know, what the hell!?

Am I awake or sleeping? I'm so tired I can't tell.

I may be crazy raving mad, I may have lost the plot.

But all this just makes me a mum to a gorgeous little tot!

Before I became a mum, I would see other mums out and about at the shops or at the park and they'd be pulling funny faces and talking goo goo gaa gaa with their babies. I'd smile to myself and think "aww bless them, they have completely lost it".

I'd always known that I wanted children and from my mid twenties, I was desperate to become a mum. However, I'd never really been around many children. So when my friends started having children, I found that I had absolutely no idea what to do or say. What do you talk about with a baby!? It doesn't talk back! At this point, I started to worry that maybe I didn't have what it took to be a mum.

Fast forward a few years and I became a mum myself. Low and behold, there I was talking goo goo gaa gaa with my own baby and thinking nothing of it. This time my husband was the one thinking I had lost it! But the truth is, I would have dressed in a clown outfit and danced around to the Macarena in the middle of the street if it meant I could hear more of her cute baby giggles (okay so maybe not in the street but you get the idea). There is nothing more magical than hearing your baby giggle and you will do whatever it takes to hear that sound over and over again.

Teething Sucks

Daddy thinks you'd win an Oscar for your constant up and down.

A gorgeous gummy grin, then tears and a frown.

A never ending waterfall of dribble down your chin.

Your top is soaking slimy wet, right through to your skin.

Your little cheeks are crimson red and raging hot to touch.

All this for just one tiny tooth but it's hurting you so much.

Now a few days of relief as we wait for number three.

This is nature's form of torture and it's so horrible to see!

For about three years during my teens, I wore all manner of braces on my teeth to sort out my fangs (yes, I had actual vampire teeth). Every few weeks, I would have to go back for them to be tightened and for several days after that I could actually feel my teeth being dragged through my gums. It hurt to chew, it hurt to swallow, it even hurt to speak. I pretty much drank a tube of Bonjela pain relief gel each day and walked around unable to feel my tongue.

I imagine this is what a teething baby must feel like...but much, much worse and for a lot, lot longer. Their cheeks are burning, their bottom is burning, they can't (won't) sleep, they produce enough snot and dribble to prevent worldwide drought and they're pretty blooming miserable. And who can blame them!

The bit about teething that the imaginary parenting manual failed to warn me about is that, for a breastfeeding woman, your boob becomes an actual teether! I think my high-pitched screams were probably heard by people from here to deepest, darkest Peru when, out of the blue, my teething baby decided to perform a crocodile death roll on my nipple!!

Pootastrophy

Oh my god it's down her legs. It's up her back. It's in her hair!

It's on the mat. It's on my hands. It's everywhere!

Do I wipe? Do I spray? Do I just stand and shout?

I don't know what to do. How did ALL this come out!?

I've always been known to stay calm in a mess.

But this is a whole new level of stress.

The clothes aren't worth saving so they're going in the bin.

Then after I've bathed her, I'm having a gin!

My first experience of baby poo was a baptism of fire. I was looking after my friend's baby boy for a couple of hours at their house whilst she went out (I won't name names as this baby is no longer a baby). Everything was going great then he toddled off into his play tent and it all went quiet. Suddenly a not-so-fragrant aroma began to waft out from inside the tent. I'd never even changed a nappy before so my immediate thought was "oh shit" (quite literally).

I bent down and tried to coax him out of the tent but he was having none of it. Then somehow he managed to sneak out through the back of the tent and I watched in horror at what unfurled. Whilst inside the tent, he must have put his hands down his nappy and there was poo everywhere. As he toddled off, he left mark after mark on everything he passed, including the sofa! He then smashed down on his bottom in the corner of the room and began to lick his fingers!!!

You'd think that this experience would have provided me with a very strong foundation for coping with pootastrophies when it came to my own baby. Yet, when that first poo up the back nappy explosion occurred, I still froze in terror like a rabbit in the headlights! I'm just thankful I was at home when it happened.

Not A Peep About Sleep

"How's the baby sleeping?" It's all people ever ask!
But I stay polite in my reply and put on a smiley mask.
"The sleep is not fantastic but we're managing just fine."
Would they really want to hear the truth and listen to me whine?
If I had the guts to do, it here's what I'd love to say:
"You moron why'd you ask me that, shut up and go away!"

In truth the baby sleeps for a short two hour block.
Then I'm sat up trying to comfort whilst looking at the clock.
I finally get her down to sleep and creep back to my bed.
Then the cycle starts all over when she wakes up to be fed.

My eyes feel really heavy, it's so hard to stay awake.
I have my toes and fingers crossed tonight we'll get a break.
I know to them it's harmless, a small question just in chat.
But it's almost like me asking "hey have you lost any fat?"

Sleep is a touchy subject, most mummies will agree.
So unless we bring the subject up, I suggest you leave it be.

I recently heard of someone in my local area offering sleep advice at a rate of £300 per night. There have been many, MANY, nights with both of my children where I would gladly have paid this amount if it meant I could close my eyes. However, I have no idea how this particular individual sleeps at night given they are, quite frankly, preying on the vulnerable!

I've lost count of the number of times people have said to me, "is she good? Does she sleep?" Sleep is good, or it would be if I had any. But I fail to understand how sleep is a measure of how "good" my baby is. Or, for that matter, how sleep determines whether I'm succeeding as a parent!

Every child is different and every night is different. Teething, developmental leaps, nightmares...they all affect sleep. So one minute you think you're winning, then out of nowhere something comes along and drags you kicking and screaming back to the start line. My eldest daughter currently has an imagination to rival Julia Donaldson meaning that there are giants, dinosaurs, goats, you name it, all in her bedroom at night, so she couldn't possibly sleep. At least not on her own anyway!

Only In It For Cake

Monday food shop, entertaining for some.

A mummy versus baby rugby scrum.

Every item of food returned in a volley.

Thank god I got the doughnuts into the trolley!

Tuesday a nice pleasant walk in the sun.

Tried to strap the hulk in...guess who won!

Baby in one arm, still pushing the pram.

Spotted a tearoom...a scone with cream and jam!

Wednesday baby yoga, a time to stretch and tone.

Babies get to sing and play whilst mummies pant and groan.

Comparing battle bruises and how long we've been awake.

Then at the end we're treated to some lovely homemade cake!

Thursday a day to tackle jobs, at least that's what I thought.

Every time I tried to leave the room, baby was distraught.

One thirty minute nap all day in which to get things done.

Instead I sat and watched TV with tea and a bun!

Friday a trip to the farm, a picnic all prepared.

I didn't take into account our picnic would be shared.

Cheese sandwich for the farmyard cat, an apple for the goat.

Good job I hid my KitKat in the pocket of my coat!

Everybody has that something that they need to get through the week. For my husband, that something is coffee. For others, it's a glass of wine or a workout. I can't stand the taste of coffee, I've never been a big drinker (well not since I left university anyway), and me and exercise just don't mix. So for me, that something is sugar! Cake, biscuits, chocolate...anything goes.

I've always had a sweet tooth but since becoming a mum, this has reached a whole new level. It's the only thing that will pull me out of the fog of sleep deprivation or pick me back up after dealing with the mother of all tantrums. I used to have a desk job working in a building that had no shop and no vending machine so there was very little in the way of cake or chocolate to tempt me. However, these days I spend my time at parks, farms, garden centres, and soft plays, all of which usually have cafes with an abundance of sweet treats on show.

I will openly admit that my sugar dependence is probably verging on addiction. I feel deprived if I've not had any all day. I know it's not good for me; I know there are healthier options but I'm sorry, an apple just doesn't cut it!

Can't Do Right

Embarrassed when they're on your boob,

but it's "second best" to give them bottle.

Feel bad to sit and take a break,

but too tired to go full throttle.

Feel guilty if you go to work,

but stay home and you're a bum.

Defeatist if you give a dummy

but don't let them suck their thumb.

You rely too much on Calpol,

but their temperature is high!?

You'll spoil them if you comfort them,

but its neglect to let them cry.

Deflated when food goes to waste,

but use a pouch and you are lazy.

Unstable if you have a cry,

but hold it in and you'll go crazy.

Can't do right for doing wrong,

but you do your very best.

Just enjoy having a little one,

and forget about the rest.

Contrary to what has seemingly been portrayed, there is no such thing as a perfect parent. As soon as you become a parent you will find that everyone, and I mean EVERYONE, will have an opinion. Your parents, your friends, health care professionals, your neighbours, another mum at a baby group, a random old man at the bus stop...they will all have something "helpful" to contribute.

I found that all of these suggestions contradicted each other and I was just left questioning every parenting decision I ever made. Is it my fault she's so clingy, do I cuddle her too much? Should I have given her a dummy, is it affecting her teeth and her speech? Should I have spoon fed her instead of doing baby led, would that have made her a less fussy eater?

The truth is there is no "correct" way to raise a child. But when I was in the thick of it, I worried myself sick that I would do something wrong which would then impact her entire future. My advice to any other parent feeling this way: cover your eyes, turn off your ears and just go with your gut (this is easier said than done, I know). But only you truly know your child and only you know what is best for them so don't let anyone take that from you!

Eat The World

How naive it was for me to think you were coming in for a kiss.
I just very nearly lost my nose, now that I think I'd miss!

Your mission is to eat the world, it seems to make you happy.
If you succeed, I dread to think of what would fill your nappy!

You're eating at the table, fist-sized chunks of juicy pear.
But then you go and crane your neck and try to taste your chair.

We're in the car I'm driving, I look in my rear view.
Your foot is right up by your face, you're chewing on your shoe.

I'm trying to sit and watch TV but the channels keep on flicking.
The remote control is in your mouth, it's getting a good licking.

"Put your money where your mouth is" must really baffle you.
But darling I did tell you, my purse is not to chew!

I know you must explore the world, it's just your way to learn.
But must you try taste everything? It makes my stomach churn!

Once my daughter had worked out how to get her fist to her mouth, that was it. Nothing was off limits! Toys, remote controls, magazines, socks, my hair! You name it, everything went in her mouth. It felt like a never-ending cycle of taking things away from her, moving them out of her reach and then watching as she found yet more things that she shouldn't be putting in her mouth...toilet paper, shoes, my phone, a plant.

She refused to be spoon fed so we went down the baby led weaning route but I was permanently on edge that something might get stuck in her throat. I would spend ages cutting up grapes and blueberries into small enough pieces so that they wouldn't be a choking hazard. Then thirty minutes later, we would be outside in the garden and I'd find her with a mouthful of gravel!

This is partly the reason why we decided to introduce a dummy. We figured that if she had a dummy in her mouth then nothing else could get in there. But as is always the case, there were those who questioned our decision. "What's she got that in her mouth for, she won't be able to talk to you." No but she won't be able to talk with a mouth full of gravel either!

Determined

My little explorer is raring to go.

I'm more than a little nervous though.

She pulls herself up to get a view from the top.

And shuffles along with the sofa as her prop.

But she can't stop now, there's a world to see.

On determined legs, she tries to run free.

She's courageous and strong so I hide my fear.

I hold out my arms and smile and cheer.

Then she falls with a crash and I feel the pain.

But she just crawls to the sofa and starts again.

From about six months old, all she wanted to do was be on her feet. She would grab our hands and pull herself up then we would be forced to walk up and down all over the house so that she could practice her steps. It killed our backs! However, we do actually have some very cute videos of her holding on to us with one hand, the other hand up in the air and her little chubby legs bopping away to Ed Sheeran. She absolutely loved to dance and still does, although her legs are slightly less chubby now.

At nine months old, she suddenly decided that she was tired of waiting for us to take her hand and walk her around - a perfect display of my patient genes coming to the surface there! She pulled herself up and set off running. Not walking, running! And she hasn't stopped since, which probably also partly explains my dependence on sugar!

It seemed like nothing was going to slow her down. Then, one day she tripped and fell smack into the door frame in our bedroom. She had a huge golf ball on her forehead with a big dent going across it in a line. I was convinced that she had cracked her skull. Thankfully she hadn't but I don't think I'd ever felt my heart race as much as it did then!

The Palatial Pigsty

I used to be quite house proud. Every item had its place.

And then a tiny meteor came crashing down from space.

There's washing hung on curtain rails. Food on every floor.

There's a bin bag full of nappies still sitting by the door.

There's no time for dusting. Just dash things down and blow.

The lawn would be a jungle if Grandad didn't come to mow.

There's a car parked in the kitchen. Its beeping horn is beeping stuck!

And we have to share our bathtub with a flashing disco duck.

A dog-sized dino by the door...it's there to meet and greet.

The sofa starts on singing when guests go to take a seat.

My scarves live in the toy box. My t-shirt in the cot.

There's tiny handprints on the windows. Every room is smeared with snot.

But we call this house our palace even with the muck and mess.

As ten months ago we welcomed our beautiful princess.

When we first moved into our house, we would spend our weekends carefully painting and decorating each room. We put a lot of hard work into getting it just right. Once the work was finished, we became quite the entertainers and enjoyed having people round. We would regularly invite friends over for dinner or a BBQ, or have people stay with us for the weekend.

Fast forward to post children and, aside from the fact that we're in bed by nine o'clock most nights, our house is a state and I would be too embarrassed to entertain anyone in it! Those carefully painted walls are now covered in scuffs where toys have been rammed into them. The patio doors are covered in snotty, yoghurty hand prints. And the carpets are, quite frankly, buggered!

For a long time, I would obsessively follow my daughter around the house, cleaning up after her, picking up toys and constantly hoovering and wiping surfaces. Then one day (probably around the time daughter number two arrived) I realised: what is the actual point! I was fighting a war I couldn't win. So these days, I just watch as they recreate a scene from Deep Impact and wait until they've gone to bed each night to start the clean up operation.

Moving On From Mummy

My heart is in my throat, I am shaking to the core.

As I walk you down the drive and knock on the door.

A smiley face to greet you, "hello baby girl".

Then I hand you on over whilst trying not to hurl.

Your face looks so confused, asking "mummy where am I?"

So as I turn and walk away, I pray that you don't cry.

They say it's worse for mummy and I hope that this is true.

As I can't do anything but sit and think of you.

I watch the minutes on the clock 'til finally you are done.

Then I rush to pick you up and hear that you've had lots of fun.

You played with other children, crawled all across the floor.

You ate up all your lunch, then went off to play some more.

An egg box was your favourite yet so many toys to choose.

And you only got upset when you needed time to snooze.

They cannot wait to have you back which makes me feel quite sad.

But you're happy, safe and having fun, for that I should be glad.

After eleven months of maternity leave, I had to go back to work. I absolutely hated my job. If anyone from my old work is reading this, I don't think this will come as a surprise! So the thought of going back and having to leave my little girl made me feel sick to my stomach. As it turned out, after taking away childcare and commuting costs, I would have made bugger all money each month anyway so we talked it over and I decided to hand in my notice.

Whilst this meant that I only had to go back for twelve weeks, we still needed childcare for this period. We decided on a local childminder and I took her there for a couple of settling in sessions prior to going back to work so that she could get used to the idea before she started going for full days.

I'm sure that any mum who's had to drop their child off at childcare for the very first time, regardless of their age, be it nursery or school, has sobbed or at least had a lump in their throat when walking away. I was a mess! But whilst I was sat worrying myself silly, she was having a whale of a time. She absolutely loved playing with all the children and didn't want to come home!

Here's To The Pre-Mum

There's so many things I used to say before I was a mum.

They've all gone out the window as most of them were dumb.

My children won't have sugar, they'll only eat the best.

Then she saw me eating cake and turned into a pest.

My children won't spend their time in front of the TV.

Let's face it that's the only way I get some time for me.

My children will be read to every single day.

But some days I just can't be bothered, OKAY!

My children won't find themselves dressed up like a dolly.

Oh this dress is pretty, let's put it in the trolley.

My children will never ever sleep in our bed.

Just sleep where you want, I feel half dead.

My children won't be spoilt with every single toy.

Then came Christmas and her birthday...oh boy.

So here's to the old me who had it all worked out.

I really didn't have a clue what it was all about!

I really wish I'd have video recorded some of the thoughts that went through my head before becoming a mum. Purely so that if I was having a bad day, I could watch it back and laugh at myself. What an uppity, naive, righteous prat I must have been!

I would see a child having a tantrum and think, "What a naughty little brat". Or I would hear parents in the supermarket bribing their children with the promise of sweets if they just behaved for a bit longer and I'd think, "Wow what a terrible way to raise your child". Honestly, anyone would think these parents had fastened chains around their child's neck and tethered them to an aeroplane given the amount of tutting that went on in my head! In fairness to my past self though, I never actually outwardly tutted anyone - it was just in my head!

I'm sure I'm not the only person who's been there done that. It is so easy to pass judgement on something you know nothing about. Last year, my eldest was in the process of potty training and was sat down on her potty next to my car in a car park when a young woman walked past, flashed a look of horror and then tutted. Oh how I wish I could have parachuted her into my life, even just for a day, to show her how much actual shit I have to deal with!

Stranger To Danger

You fire round the house like you're riding a rocket.

Feed toys and your fingers into every socket.

You swing on the curtains like you belong in a zoo.

Head first off the sofa and the bed too.

You climb up the stairs like there's a fox on your tail.

Try eat every stone, twig, beetle and snail.

Bump your head, graze your knees, you scream out in pain.

Then the next day you do it all over again.

You're a stranger to danger, there's no fear in sight.

But knock ten years off my life from fright after fright!

When I came home from hospital with my newborn baby, it was as though everything had suddenly become a hazard overnight. What if I fall down the stairs whilst I'm holding her? What if I trip up whilst pushing the pram and it rolls off down the hill? What if the ceiling light suddenly falls down and lands on her? You can laugh but that last one actually happened to me when we were living in our last rented house.

I think it's fair to say that I'm quite an overprotective, overly cautious parent. I can't help it, I see danger everywhere. So as this tiny baby turned into a headstrong toddler, a battle of wills began. Where I saw danger, she saw fun. And the word NO just encouraged her to do it even more! As she's grown, I've learnt to pick my battles and I've slackened my grip slightly. Only slightly. She's now allowed to go on the climbing frame at the park by herself.

Me, my brother and sister used to always laugh at my mum for how protective she was over us as children. One Christmas, Santa brought us all rollerblades...along with a helmet, knee pads, elbow pads and wrist guards. If either of my two get rollerblades, they'll be wearing an inflatable sumo man costume every time they use them! God help me if one of them decides they want to be a racing car driver when they're older!

Love You More

You're a little person now and you're learning every day,

What to say and do to try and get your way.

Saying I-YAAAA to everybody on the street.

Raiding kitchen cupboards for more food to eat.

If your actions make us giggle, you go again and again.

Your funny choo choo hand wave to signal a train.

You're hysteric every time we chase you round and roar.

"Let's go out" and in seconds you're stood waiting by the door.

You've given up on nap times, now a 13 hour day.

Five minutes and you've lost interest so that's a lot of games to play!

You've added to your dance moves, a twirl and a kick.

But you're never ever happy with the music that we pick.

When I held you as a newborn just listening to you snore.

I really didn't think that I could love you more.

Yes it's been a challenge and each day brings something new.

But there's nothing in this world I wouldn't give up for you.

My husband refers to this rhyme as soppy but you can't write a book about being a parent without at least one soppy section. Because let's face it, no matter how much trouble they cause and no matter how much they keep you awake at night, they still have a way of wrapping you right around their little finger! If my husband forgets to take the bin out to the street, I'll be pissed off at him for a week. My daughter could sling horse poo in my face and all would be forgiven within thirty minutes.

It's hard to explain the love you feel for your child. It's completely different to the love you feel towards a partner or a friend. It's unconditional and it never fades, regardless of whether they're right there with you or a million miles away.

It sounds silly but the feelings I had for my daughter straight after she was born took me completely by surprise. They were overwhelming. I didn't think it was possible to love her more than I did when she was first here. But as her little personality started to grow, so did my love for her. So much so that when I fell pregnant the second time, I worried I might not have any room left to love another child. But I'm glad to say I was very wrong!

Sick Of Being Sick

Right now I'm rocking scratty hair and a grubby, too big sweater.

An improvement on last weeks look as we're finally feeling better.

I always used to hear it said "they're a magnet for all germs".

Well my magnet is a strong one, in no uncertain terms!

She picks up every illness going and I fall right behind.

Another stint in quarantine and I think I'll lose my mind!

I now have lots of nightmares about a giant ten-armed bug.

It slides into the ball pool and looks at me all smug.

"It's good for her immune system, germs will make her stronger."

She'll soon have strength to rival Thor if she's sick for any longer!

You'd think that having hyperemesis during my pregnancy would have stood me in good stead for the amount of sick involved with having a small child. Nope! The evil lurgies that cause sickness in small children are everywhere. They're relentless and spare no one!! Siblings, parents, grandparents, friends...no one is safe. All you can do is dose up on vitamins and hope for the best. Either that or just never do anything or see anyone.

At the time of writing this rhyme, we'd had a particularly bad run of sickness. It was the autumn/winter after my daughter turned one. First it was a cold, then a stomach bug, then flu, then a stomach bug, then the bloody Aussie flu! We barely had time to recover from one illness before we were struck down by the next. We barely left the house and yet somehow, the lurgies still managed to find us.

My husband had taken so much time off work that they were threatening to refer him to occupational health. I'm not entirely sure what they could have done to help him though. Perhaps they could have offered to pay for us to stay in an isolation unit for the rest of the winter?

It's Okay To Say I'm Not Okay

There are good days, there are bad days and many days in between.

There are days I laugh my head off and days I want to scream.

There are days when I get so damn tired of picking up all her stuff.

There are days when I do wonder whether all this is enough.

There are days she finally works things out and I do a little jig.

There are days I want to strangle those who created Peppa Pig.

There are days I feel so lonely and I don't know what to do.

There are days I really need a break so I go sit on the loo.

It's okay to say I'm not okay. It's okay if I feel glum.

It doesn't mean I'm undeserving or make me a rubbish mum.

I always find it very difficult reading this rhyme because at the time of writing it, I was not okay. Even as I write this now, three years later, my eyes are filling up. And yet, the message I convey in the rhyme is so hypocritical because I didn't tell a single person, not even my husband.

I was so desperately lonely and felt like I'd lost my identity and self worth. I remember reading a post on social media that said, "Comment below with your favourite song at the moment" and I just burst into tears. I had no idea what music I liked as all I'd heard for the last few weeks was the theme tune to Peppa flipping Pig! Every day I would achieve nothing and every night my husband would come home and I'd have absolutely nothing to tell him.

Becoming a stay-at-home mum was my choice. I left a job that I had trained for years to get. Was it the right decision for our family? One hundred percent! But I truly believed that if I opened up about how I was feeling, the general consensus from everyone around me would be, "It was your choice: you're very lucky to have even had the option, so stop your whinging". And in some ways I was right to believe this because, when I did finally start to talk about things, there was more than just one person who thought that going and getting a job would solve all my worries.

Little

Little fingers in my ears, in my eyes and up my nose.

Little hands wiping food and snot down my clothes.

Little legs you disappear on in the blink of an eye.

Little feet you stomp in anger and kick whilst you cry.

Little arms you hold out when you're seeking a hug.

Little head on my chest all sleepy and snug.

Little smile makes my stern face completely fall apart.

Little lady there's no doubt you will always have my heart.

Something I have heard my mum say quite a few times now is, "You forget how little they were". This always makes me feel quite sad because, whilst my children are still little, I know exactly what she means. It is so easy to get caught up in just getting through each day, each week, each month that time suddenly passes you by. Recently, I have been trying to make a conscious effort to stand back and soak up their littleness a bit more but it isn't always easy with everything going on.

The morning after our second daughter was born, our eldest came running in and it was as though she had doubled in size overnight. No it wasn't because her grandparents had fattened her up with treats whilst we were in hospital, although they probably did. In actual fact, she hadn't grown at all. But holding this tiny newborn baby in my arms, my eldest no longer seemed "little".

Next year she will be starting school and I'm already questioning whether I have made the most of having her at home with me. It seems to have just crept up on us from out of nowhere. It won't be long before she is packing her bags and leaving home, and I'll be left grieving for the little girl she once was.

A Feud With Food

There was a battle with the bolognese.

Weetabix caused a war!

She threw her food across the table

then started screaming "I want more!"

Utter carnage with the custard.

The fish pie picked a fight.

But if she goes to bed still hungry

then she'll wake up in the night.

Hostility over hot cross buns.

An apple went under attack.

She'll refuse all food I give her

then ask me for a snack!

The clash of titans over casserole.

The rice is in retreat.

I'm so tired of all the struggles

so please just fricking eat!

When we were growing up, we used to walk into the kitchen when my mum was cooking and ask, "What's for tea mum" and she would reply, "Wait and see tea". This basically meant that we weren't going to like the meal and she knew it. Between the three of us she probably used this phrase almost every day because she could never please all of us with anything she cooked.

She adopted this approach to try and delay the whinging from us all when we found out what we were having to eat. However, it didn't take us very long to see straight through her tactics and the whinging resumed. Wow we were annoying!

Now I'm a mum to an extremely fussy eater myself and it is, quite simply, soul destroying. I will spend ages preparing a freshly cooked meal for it to be strewn across the dinner table before she has even picked up her fork and tried it! One day she tells me she likes carrots and I rejoice that she finally likes something that contains vitamins. Then the next day she tells me that carrots are "gusty".

I try to take solace from the fact that me, my brother and my sister no longer survive on jam sandwiches alone so we must have grown out of the fussy eating at some point. However, it doesn't make it any less frustrating right now!

Mum Friends

Being a mum is not that easy.

You can often feel alone.

All your old friends are out working

so they can't answer the phone.

So you need to make some mum friends

who are going through it too.

Some friends you can send photos

with "is this a normal poo?"

Other mums think nothing of it

when you break down and weep.

They're awake during the night

and slur their words through lack of sleep.

You'll share laughter over leaky boobs

and failing pelvic floors.

You'll take comfort knowing each of them

are fighting similar wars.

Other mums know the importance

of coffee, cake and wine.

They can see straight through the lies

when you say "I am fine!"

If it wasn't for your children

you may never have met.

But friendships formed through motherhood

are ones you won't forget.

During the second half of my pregnancy, I was very fortunate to be able to attend pregnancy yoga and antenatal classes. I was even more lucky to have the same amazing teacher for both classes who was great at fostering friendships between the mums to be. It meant that I left both these classes having exchanged phone numbers with two separate groups of women.

We were all different ages, came from different backgrounds and had chosen different career paths. A few of these women, like me, were expecting their first baby; others were expecting their second. But the one thing we all had in common, regardless of these differences, is that we were all expecting a baby at around the same time.

All of these women have been there for me in some shape or form since the birth of my eldest, sharing advice and support; cheering me on when I've completely lost all faith in my ability to raise a child; arranging much needed meet-ups with and without children; even just providing a forum in which I could have a whine and a moan. Ladies, you know who you are - thank you so much for everything. I would never have come this far without you!

Fear Of Soft Play

Soft play. Now there's two words I dread.

Thinking of all those germs that are spread.

Not a time to relax and drink my tea.

As I'm too busy being a child referee.

Parents look at you and give you 'the eye'.

Trying to work out if you're friendly or shy.

All shouting "move away from the end of that slide"

And watching them drown in a ball pool tide.

Then there's always that child who will push and kick.

And another one with endless bogies to pick.

"Why go there then?" I hear you all say.

Well it's better than being in the house all day!

If you'd not already gathered from my rhyme, I HATE soft play! For those of you who haven't had the delight yet, let me set the scene...

It's a cold, wet, miserable day. It has been a cold, wet, miserable day every day for the past week! We've exhausted every possible activity in the house and my toddler is now climbing the walls so I bundle her into the car and drive to a soft play in the hope that she'll burn off some energy whilst I sit and drink a cup of coffee.

We get there and she refuses to go in without me. Goodbye coffee! I clamber up the levels, squeezing through rollers and the tiniest holes ever. We finally make it to the slide, we sit down and she says, "No I'm too scared". We make the same journey but in reverse back down the levels and head to the ball pool where I'm forced to submerge myself alongside another child who has just sneezed all over the balls. Oh and just to further point out the cleanliness of these ball pools, I recently lost my milk-soaked breast pad in one, never to be seen again!

We finally call it a day, get back in the car and she falls fast asleep on the journey home. So whilst she's recharging her batteries ready to resume climbing the walls, I feel like I've just had a full workout and need to lie down!

Second Shadow

She "helps" me when I'm cooking. She "helps" me wash the pots.

She "helps" me put my trainers on by tying them in knots.

She's there when I am sleeping. She's there when I get dressed.

She's there to do my makeup and ensure I "look my best."

She's with me on the toilet. She's with me when I shower.

She's with me every minute of every single hour.

I have a second shadow. On rare occasions it breaks free.

But just like Peter Pan, without my shadow I'm not me.

I think one of the things I find the hardest about being a mum is that I have very little time to myself. I wake up in the morning and my eldest is right there. Either she's in our bed after a horrific night or she's stood by the side of our bed right next to my head, waiting for me to open my eyes. I climb out of bed and she follows me to the toilet. She insists on coming in the shower with me, then sits next to me by the mirror when I do my makeup. And it pretty much continues like this for the rest of the day until she goes to bed.

In some ways it's quite cute having a little sidekick and seeing how much she looks up to me. But then when she's stood banging on the bathroom door crying because I've locked it and she wants to come in, I just feel like shouting, "For gods sake I just want to poo in peace!"

Being a stay at home mum probably intensifies this further as I never get a break from them and likewise, they never get a break from me. But then when I do go out without them, just for a meal or to see a movie, I feel ridiculously guilty that I've left them! Which is very silly I know because at the end of the day, if I don't look after myself, I can't look after them and everyone deserves a break.

Mummy Who?

When I first took her to childcare, she would stick to me like glue.

She didn't want to leave me. I felt the same way too.

As they prised my baby off me, her arms still reaching out,

Her big eyes looked so sad and "Mama" she would shout.

With a big smile on my face, I waved and said goodbye.

Then I'd get back in my car and cry and cry and cry.

Now it's ten months later and she clearly loves it there.

This morning when I said goodbye, she really didn't care.

She snatched her bag from in my hand and ran straight for the door.

She pushed past other parents and threw her bag onto the floor.

Then off she went, no looking back, to find her friends and play.

She doesn't want or need me now, it's another sad, sad day!

This follows on quite nicely from the last section about having time to myself. After I'd finished my notice period at work, rather than just pulling our daughter back out of childcare, we decided to keep sending her one day a week. She had settled in so well with the childminder and we both felt it would be good for her to continue mixing with other children without me there as her security blanket. Plus, it meant that I then had one day a week where I could get on with things without her at my feet.

The first few times I dropped her off she understandably got quite upset. After a while, things improved as she came to understand that I wasn't going to drop her off and abandon her there for good. We would go in, have a kiss and a cuddle, I'd say "have a good day darling" and she'd wave goodbye.

Then one day, she ditched the kiss and the cuddle, and didn't even say goodbye. She just walked off! It felt like time had suddenly jumped and she was a thirteen-year-old wanting nothing more to do with me. I dread the day that she no longer finds my silly antics funny and I just become one big embarrassment in front of her friends.

Please Just Bring Me Wine

So these tantrums she keeps having…what are they about!?

She's got such a little temper and wow she can shout!

One minute she is playing, the next all hell breaks loose.

Surely this is classed as poor parent abuse?

She lays down in public and proceeds to punch the floor.

Her body goes all rigid when I say "you can't have more".

She'll have wrinkles like a Basset if she keeps up with this frown.

And god help me if I dare to say "just calm down".

What's happened to my child because this one isn't mine.

Can anyone, just someone please just bring me wine!

Before I became a mum, if you'd have asked any of my close friends or family to describe me in three words, "patient" would not have been one of them. Yet somehow, the one thing that I've been commended on the most as a mum is how patient I am with my children. Or at least I was until the terrible twos hit!

One minute she was the same loving little girl she'd always been. Then out of nowhere, it was like she'd been possessed by some sort of prehistoric fish. She would throw herself down and begin flapping and flailing around on the floor whilst roaring and screeching at the top of her voice. I just couldn't keep up with her mood swings and I soon found myself tiptoeing around, trying not to do anything that might set her off again.

The first few times this happened, I tried talking her down and ended up raising my voice at her. Then I realised that there's no point trying to reason with a dinosaur and decided that the best thing to do was to just walk away and leave her to calm down. This worked a treat at home but it's not that easy to just walk away from your child in the middle of a supermarket. Instead, I would drag her kicking and screaming to the wine aisle!

Snuggles

She's fallen asleep on me watching TV.

Her mouth is wide open, as cute as can be.

There's so many jobs that I need to do.

Making dinner and washing to name just two.

I really should go lay her down in her cot.

But how could I possibly move from this spot?

When she's awake, she's go, go, go!

Always top speed with no time to slow.

So sod the jobs, I really don't care.

This time is precious and these snuggles are rare.

Growing up, if ever we were sick, hurt or upset, my mum would give us a little cuddle and tell us we'd be alright. But we were never the kind of family that just cuddled for cuddles sake. In fact, if either of my parents came to me now and gave me a hug, I'd probably panic thinking they had some awful news to tell me.

I've probably gone to the other extreme with my children. I cuddle them all the time both at home and in public. I cuddle them when they're sad or when they're happy, to acknowledge an apology when they've been a handful, to say well done I'm proud of you, or for absolutely no reason whatsoever. We love nothing more than cuddling up on the sofa together under a blanket and watching a movie.

I know that there's an old school of thought that you can "spoil" your child by holding them too much but to be honest, I don't actually know what "spoiling a child" even means! All I know is that, when either of my girls come to me and give me a cuddle or say "I love you mummy", no matter how bad a day I've had, it always makes me feel happy. So in my mind, if they get the same feeling from me when I show them affection then why would I not!?

Don't Tell A Mummy How To Mummy

Every mummy wants to be the best mummy they can be.

But there's no such thing as perfect, every mummy will agree.

Be a relative or stranger, it's not your place to say.

You need to let each mummy find her own mummy way.

A child that's fed and happy, be it bottle or breast.

Is a child with a mummy who is doing what is best.

A child may suck their thumb or they may have a dummy.

But it's no one else's business so just leave it to the mummy.

If a child is in a tantrum and falls down on their butt.

It's a hard day for the mummy so don't stand there and tut.

That child needs putting down more, that child eats too much food.

Whatever you are thinking, don't say it, it's just rude!

Don't tell a mummy how to mummy, she's doing her very best.

And your small piece of "advice" may just leave that mummy stressed.

I've lost count of the number of times I've received unwanted parenting advice. It's not so bad if it's from someone who actually knows you. But why is it that complete strangers feel that it's okay to approach you in the street and share their wisdom!? Had I been on my own, they would probably have walked straight past me without even giving me a second glance.

On one occasion, I was queuing to pay in a shop and my baby was crying in her pram. A woman came up to me, put her hand on my shoulder in the most patronising way and said, "I think you're baby needs feeding love". Oh thank you so much for pointing that out; I'd never have known otherwise!

On another occasion, we were at the park with my little girl toddling around and a woman approached me to say, "There's a chill in the air so that child should have a hat on". If only she knew the battles I'd fought trying to get a bloody hat on her head!

With both of these women, I just smiled awkwardly and said nothing. I hate confrontation and I've never been able to come up with something witty on the spot in these types of situations. It means that I always walk away feeling extremely irritated and start running through all the things I should have said in my head.

Lub You

This little blonde parrot copies everything I say.

She repeated my swear word just the other day.

The TV wasn't working so she shouted "nob-ed".

Daddy didn't hear it. If he had, I'd be dead!

Banana is a "naaana". Every cup she sees is "tea".

It's a long walk through the woods when she points out every tree.

Every doggy gets a "woof". Every baby gets an "awww".

And wow do I hate the words "more, more, more".

She's really quite polite. She always says "yeh pease".

And when I say we're going out she reminds me I need "keee's".

A self-proclaimed "good girl" even when she's really not.

When she doesn't want her food she claims that it's too "ot".

This evening as it reached the time for her to say "na-night",

I tucked her into bed and turned off the light.

Then through the dark I heard her say "mummy lub you".

And trying not to cry I said "I love you too".

Our eldest was an extremely early walker. We had kind of expected it as she'd been desperate to move right from the get-go. Her speech, however, was somewhat slower to develop. Looking back, it was probably just because her brain was so busy working on her movement or perhaps that she had no need to communicate because she could get up and get things for herself without having to ask. Nevertheless, we were still concerned at how slowly her words were coming.

As a parent, it's extremely difficult to stop yourself from comparing your child to others of a similar age. Most of her little friends were talking in broken sentences already whilst we struggled to get more than a handful of words out of her. We were told by friends, family and other parents, "Don't worry they all catch up" but this didn't stop us from worrying.

As it turned out, all of them were right. It was almost as though she just figured everything out in her sleep one night and then woke up the next day with verbal diarrhoea. She went from hardly saying anything to hardly staying quiet. And she hasn't stopped talking since. I guess it's just like the age-old saying...be careful what you wish for!

Being A Mummy

Being a mummy means learning a whole new way to share.

It means choosing time for eating or time to do your hair.

Being a mummy means never ever, ever, EVER being alone.

It means each day is an adventure into the great unknown.

Being a mummy means to juggle as though you have ten hands.

It means forever saying no to unreasonable demands.

Being a mummy means to worry that you're never good enough.

It means clinging on to sanity when your day has been so rough.

Being a mummy means to cheerlead for the smallest little thing.

It means being a dinosaur, a horse or a human swing.

Being a mummy means to laugh and cry and then to laugh some more.

It means you feel love like you never have before.

Above all else, being a mummy means to encourage and inspire.

And to hope no matter what you do, you're a mummy to admire.

It seems obvious to say but becoming a parent is so much more than a change of name (if you're not already aware, you will find yourself referred to as Mummy or Daddy more than any other name from now on). You don't just take on one new persona, you have to adopt multiple different ones all at once - carer, teacher, entertainer, chef, bogie wiper. And each one of these brings its own challenges.

Reading back through what I have written, it has been quite an eye opener to see just how many times I have mentioned my own mum. Right from being a teenager I have always said, "I will not raise my children the way my mum raised me". I'm sure most people have said this at some point in their lives but I was adamant.

What I have since come to realise is that, whilst I may not have agreed with every decision she made, she was simply doing what she thought was best at the time. And at the end of the day, that is all any parent can do.

So if you take anything from this book, please take comfort in the knowledge that we're all "failing", we all have good and bad days and, regardless of what others say, we're all doing a blooming fantastic job!

Thank You!

Firstly, thank you so much for buying the book and for reading this far! I really hope you found it enjoyable and can take something from what I have written. But I haven't achieved any of this on my own.

When others have told me it can't be done, my husband has been the one saying, "Yes it can!" I will never be able to thank him enough for his love and encouragement. And let's face it, without him I'd never have had any content for this book!

To my parents and parents-in-law, thank you for laying the foundations for us as parents and for all the love and support you continue to show us and our girls.

To Lisa, Georgie, Alice, Lauren, Claire and Rebecca, thank you all for providing such great sounding boards and for putting up with me babbling on about these rhymes for the last three and a bit years!

Finally, thank you to everyone who has contributed to this book in any way, shape or form, be it inspiration, proofreading, encouragement or support. I couldn't have done it without you.